THE STROKE SURVIVOR HANDBOOK

THE STROKE SURVIVOR HANDBOOK

Brian Maram

Copyright

No part of this publication may be reproduced, distributed, or transmitted in any form or by any means, including photocopying, recording, or other electronic or mechanical methods, without the prior written permission from the copyright holder., except in the case of brief quotations embodied in critical reviews and certain other non-commercial uses permitted by copyright law.

The Author has made every effort to trace and acknowledge sources/resources/individuals. In the event that any images/information have been incorrectly attributed or credited, the Author will be pleased to rectify these omissions at the earliest opportunity

For permission requests, email the copyright holder at the address below:

Email: info@neuvare.com

Author Page: www.amazon.com/author/brianmaram

Author Website: www.brianmaram.neuvare.com

Publisher: www.neuvare.com

Book Cover by: Brian Maram

Second edition: 2024

Copyright © 2024 Brian Maram
All rights reserved.
ISBN: 9798227590886

Dedication

To the doctors, therapists, and nurses whose unwavering dedication and compassion bring hope to stroke survivors and their families.
Your skill, patience, and kindness transform lives each day, guiding patients through their most challenging journeys.
Thank you for the strength and care you bring to every step of recovery.

Disclaimer

This book is a work of non-fiction intended to provide accurate information on the subject matter discussed. The content is based on factual information provided to and by the author, any similarities to real, fictional, or historical individuals, living or deceased, are purely coincidental.

This book is not intended to diagnose or treat any medical conditions. For diagnosis or treatment of any health concerns, please consult a qualified physician. The author, editor, and publisher are not responsible for any specific health or allergy needs that may require medical supervision and are not liable for any damages or negative consequences arising from any treatments, actions, applications, or preparations related to the information in this book. This book should not be considered a substitute for professional medical advice. Readers are encouraged to regularly consult a physician, especially in cases of symptoms requiring diagnosis or medical attention.

Based on the author's personal experience, this book is designed to provide information and motivation to its readers. It is sold with the understanding that the author, editor and publisher are not providing medical, psychological, legal, or any other professional advice. The content reflects the personal views and opinions of the author. Neither the author, editor, nor publisher shall be held liable for any physical, psychological, emotional, financial, or commercial damages, including, but not limited to, special, incidental, or consequential damages. You are responsible for your own choices, actions, and results.

The author, editor and publisher disclaim any liability for any loss, damage, or disruption caused by errors or omissions in the information, whether due to negligence, accident, or any other cause.

Preface

If you're picking up this book, it's likely that you or someone close to you has faced the intense, life-altering impact of a stroke. The initial relief of survival often masks the complex and turbulent journey that lies ahead. While there may be joy in knowing your loved one has pulled through, few are truly prepared for the reality of what comes next.

Your loved one has cleared the first hurdle by surviving, but now the real challenge begins—a challenge that will test everyone's resilience and adaptability. Life as you once knew it will change dramatically, opening up a future that neither you nor your family could ever have anticipated. With no manual to guide you through these turbulent waters, you'll find yourselves improvising, learning with each unexpected twist and turn.

The author, himself a stroke survivor, experienced a devastating brainstem haemorrhage in the pons region and was given just a 2% chance of surviving those critical early hours. From that day forward, his family's world was turned upside down in ways they could never have imagined. No one was prepared for the overwhelming range of emotions that would emerge. As brain cells began to die from a lack of oxygen, his behaviour and personality began to shift, posing some of the most difficult adjustments for both him and his family.

This book provides insight and understanding into the journey that follows a stroke—a journey that may last months or even years. It is a resource to help you prepare for the complex path ahead.

Acknowledgements

I would like to thank my children, as well as the doctors, therapists, and nurses, whose dedicated help and support made this book possible. Thank you for your patience and guidance.

About the Author

The authors life took an unexpected turn at 46 when a devastating stroke in 2011 reshaped his world.

Navigating the physical and emotional aftermath of stroke, largely on his own, the author intimately understood the daily unspoken struggles that both survivors and caregivers face. He experienced firsthand the immense burden placed on unprepared family members, many of whom navigate the demanding 24/7 caregiving role without any guidance.

The complexities only deepened when narcissism entered the mix, turning an already challenging situation into an emotional battleground.

With little support and an uncertain future, he found healing through journaling.

Determined to share his hard-earned wisdom, the authors debut book—The Stroke Survivor HandBook—was first published in 2016. A simple act that blossomed into a new passion as an author, and he now dedicates his writing to offering practical advice, emotional support, and hope to stroke survivors, caregivers, and those dealing with narcissism.

His books are a lifeline for anyone facing these trials, providing readers with the tools to navigate their toughest moments and find strength in the face of adversity.

Table of Contents

Brain Anatomy

The brain is the most complex organ within the human body. It governs all other organs, processes sensory input, and makes thought, emotions, and memory possible.

With around 86 billion neurons connected by trillions of synapses, it creates intricate networks for various functions, from language, to movement, to decision-making, and complex reasoning.

Anatomy

The brain is divided into three principal regions, consisting of the Cerebrum, Cerebellum and the Brainstem. Each handling specialised tasks, but all work together through a highly coordinated system.

The brain is also responsible for regulating involuntary functions such as heartbeat and breathing, illustrating its role as the body's ultimate control centre.

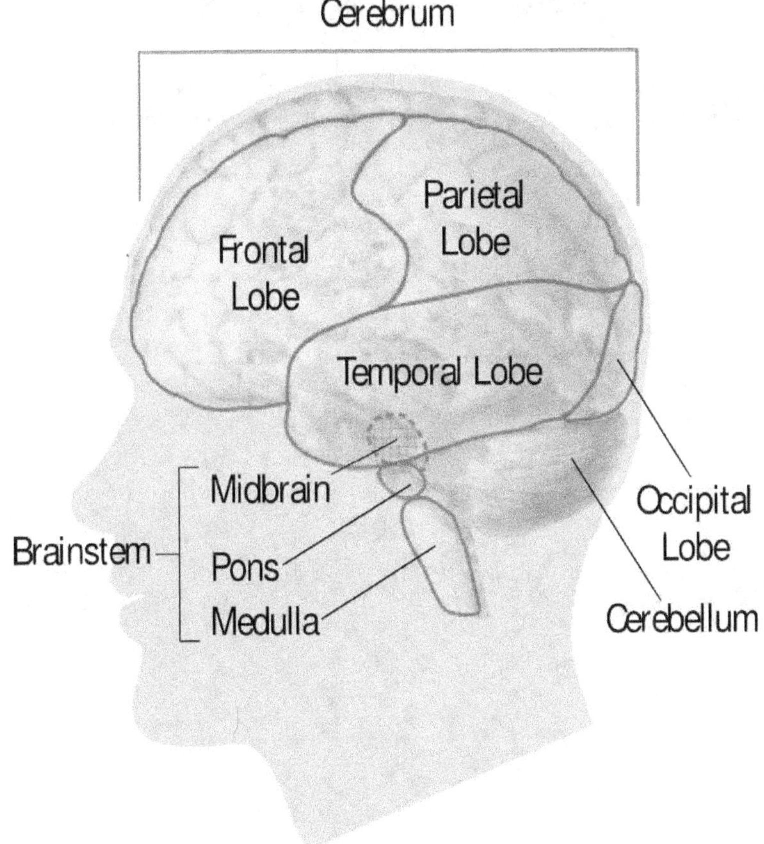

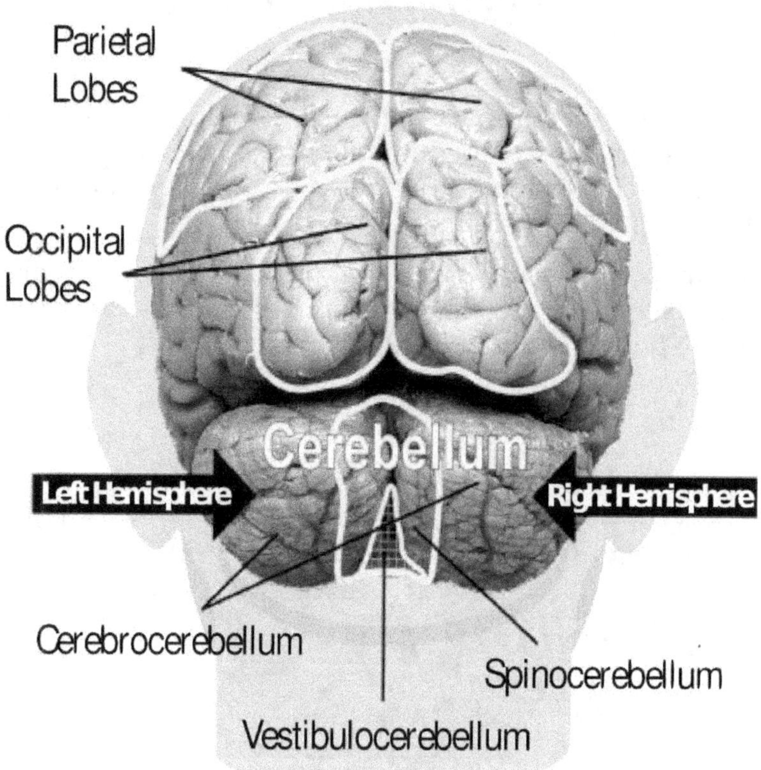

Parietal Lobes
Occipital Lobes
Cerebellum
Left Hemisphere
Right Hemisphere
Cerebrocerebellum
Spinocerebellum
Vestibulocerebellum

Cerebrum

The cerebrum is the brain's largest region, which is split into two hemispheres—the left and right cerebral hemispheres—linked by a network of nerve fibres known as the corpus callosum. These hemispheres contain four main lobes: the frontal, temporal, parietal, and occipital lobes, each of which houses substructures responsible for specific tasks.

Key functions of the cerebrum include:

Processing sensory input from the eyes, ears, skin, and other sense organs.

Coordinating voluntary actions, such as walking, talking, and writing.

Overseeing cognitive abilities like reasoning, planning, emotional responses, problem-solving, and memory.

Handling language comprehension and production.

Each hemisphere controls and interprets signals from the opposite side of the body which are essential to daily life.

The cerebrum plays a central role in virtually all our daily functions.

Damage to the cerebrum can lead to a variety of impairments such as motor dysfunction, sensory disturbances, speech and language difficulties, memory and cognitive issues, emotional and behavioural changes, vision problems, seizures, coordination and balance.

Frontal Lobe

The frontal lobes are located at the front of the brain and comprise the largest portion of the cerebral cortex. They serve as the primary site for higher cognitive functioning.

The substructures that make up the frontal lobe include the prefrontal cortex, orbitofrontal cortex, motor and premotor cortices, Broca's area, frontal eye fields, and the middle and inferior frontal gyri.

Functions associated with the frontal lobe play a significant role in voluntary movement. Activities such as walking are controlled by the primary motor cortex located within this lobe. Other functions encompass executive processes such as decision-making, planning, problem-solving, judgment, inhibition, and critical thinking; attention and thought; voluntary behaviour; cognition; intelligence; language processing and comprehension; among many others.

Damage to the frontal lobe can lead to paralysis, mood changes, and atypical social behaviours or personality changes.

Individuals may experience emotions that are not necessarily expressed through their facial expressions or voice. Conversely, they may also display excessive emotional reactions.

Parietal Lobe

The substructures that make up the parietal lobe include the somatosensory cortex, inferior and superior parietal lobules, and the precuneus.

Functions associated with the parietal lobe include the perception and integration of somatosensory information (such as touch, pressure, pain, and temperature), visuospatial processing, spatial attention and mapping, as well as number representation.

Damage to the parietal lobe can lead to an inability to locate and recognise objects, hemispatial neglect, disorientation, and a lack of coordination.

Temporal Lobe

The temporal lobe consists of several substructures, including the amygdala, primary auditory cortex, superior and middle temporal gyri, Wernicke's area, and the fusiform gyrus.

Functions associated with the temporal lobe include perception (hearing, vision, and smell), face recognition, learning and memory, understanding language, and emotional reactions.

Damage to the temporal lobe may result in difficulties in understanding speech (Wernicke's aphasia), recognising faces and objects, the inability to attend to sensory input, persistent talking, memory loss (both short- and long-term), changes in sexual behaviour, increased aggression, and difficulty recalling visual stimuli.

Temporal lobe dysfunction is closely linked to the neuropathology of schizophrenia.

Occipital Lobe

The two occipital lobes are the smallest among the four pairs of lobes in the cerebral cortex. The primary visual area of the brain is located in the occipital cortex.

As the main centre for vision, it contains most of the anatomical regions of the visual cortex, and its substructures include the cuneus and visual areas V1 to V5.

The occipital lobe is primarily associated with vision, and damage to this area may result in hallucinations, blindness, and an inability to perceive colour or motion.

Cerebellum

The Cerebellum is located at the brain's posterior and is positioned under the cerebrum hemispheres.

It is the region of the brain responsible for coordinating and regulating motor behaviour, particularly automatic movements.

Functions associated with the cerebellum include voluntary movement, motor learning, reflexes, balance, posture, timing, and sequence learning.

Damage to this area of the brain may result in a loss of coordination, tremors, an inability to walk, dizziness (vertigo), or slurred speech.

Brainstem

The brainstem is situated in the posterior part of the brain and serves as a continuation of the spinal cord. It is composed of structures that lie deep within the brain, including the pons, medulla oblongata, and midbrain. The brainstem plays a vital role in maintaining and controlling involuntary functions such as blood pressure, breathing, heartbeat, digestion, perspiration, and temperature regulation, as well as alertness, sleep, balance, and the startle response.

It also acts as a crucial relay centre, transmitting signals between the brain and the rest of the body, and is involved in regulating alertness, sleep cycles, and motor control.

Given its importance, damage to the brainstem can have severe and wide-ranging effects on the body's basic functions and overall health.

Together, these three structures—the pons, medulla oblongata, and midbrain—form the brainstem, which maintains vital processes, integrates sensory and motor functions and supports essential life-sustaining actions.

Pons

The pons plays a crucial role in relaying signals between different parts of the brain and is responsible for regulating key bodily functions. The Latin word pons means "bridge," which is fitting, as it acts as a "bridge" connecting the cerebrum and cerebellum. This connection allows for the transmission of signals between various regions of the brain, facilitating coordination, balance, and communication among these structures. The pons is also responsible for controlling breathing rhythms and contributes to functions such as sleep, arousal, and facial sensation.

Damage to the pons is life-threatening and requires urgent medical intervention. It can lead to serious impairments such as breathing and respiratory issues, movement and coordination problems, paralysis or weakness, sensory deficits, facial muscle weakness and sleep disturbances.

Medulla Oblongata

The medulla oblongata is essential for regulating involuntary bodily functions vital for sustaining life, including heart rate, blood pressure, and respiratory rate. It serves as a primary control centre for autonomic functions, ensuring that the body's internal environment remains stable. Additionally, the medulla oblongata houses reflex centres that manage actions such as swallowing, coughing, and sneezing, helping to protect respiratory and cardiovascular stability.

The medulla oblongata is where the left side of the brain crosses over to control the right side of the body, and the right side crosses over to control the left side. This crossover occurs at a point known as the decussation of the pyramids, where the nerve fibres from each hemisphere intersect. This arrangement explains why an injury to one side of the brain can impact motor skills and sensory functions on the opposite side of the body.

Damage to the medulla oblongata can be extremely serious and even life-threatening. This region of the brainstem can cause respiratory issues, cardiovascular problems, difficulty swallowing (Dysphagia), impaired gag and cough reflexes, speech and vocal Issues.

Midbrain

The midbrain functions as a relay station for auditory and visual information, integrating sensory signals and controlling eye movement, motor coordination, and reflexes related to vision and hearing. It also contains the reticular formation, which influences alertness, and the substantia nigra, a structure essential for movement, reward, and addiction. Although part of the midbrain, the substantia nigra is functionally connected with the basal ganglia, which is situated within the cerebral hemispheres and plays a crucial role in regulating movement through its production of dopamine.

Damage to the midbrain can lead to significant consequences due to its role in regulating eye movements, processing auditory and visual information, maintaining alertness, and coordinating motor functions.

Understanding Stroke

*Survivors may ramble on about things that are out of the norm.
Listen to the survivor and believe what they are telling you.*

Types of Strokes

In the unpredictability of life, stroke normally strikes unexpectedly with little to no warning. In a split second partners become caregivers and bread winners become unemployable.

Finding yourself trapped in the world of a stroke survivor can be daunting for both the survivors and those close to them.

Typically, one of two types of stroke may occur. In both cases the brain is deprived of vital oxygen, causing cells to die. Depending on the severity and damage caused, the aftermath can be overwhelming.

Ischaemic strokes account for about 80% of strokes. They are painless and caused by a blockage or clot referred to as a thrombus or an embolus. These blockages obstruct blood flow to the brain.

A thrombus develops inside a blood vessel, whereas an embolus originates elsewhere in the body and moves to obstruct blood flow to the brain.

Haemorrhagic strokes on the other hand are less common and account for about 20% of strokes. They are characterised by a sudden and severe sharp pain which occurs at a time when a blood vessel ruptures, causing bleeding within the brain.

Transient Ischaemic Attack (TIA)

Transient Ischemic Attacks (TIAs), often referred to as "mini-strokes," share similar symptoms with strokes but are typically short-lived, usually lasting less than 24 hours.

Unlike strokes, TIAs do not cause brain cell death, meaning they do not result in permanent disabilities. Although painless, they should never be ignored.

It is essential to take TIAs seriously and seek medical attention, as they can signal a heightened risk of a more severe stroke in the future.

Stroke Prevention

Adopt a proactive approach to managing health and lifestyle factors that contribute to stroke risk. Below is a list of ten common contributing factors:

1. High Blood Pressure
2. Diabetes
3. Maintain a Healthy Diet
4. Stay Physically Active
5. Quit Smoking
6. Limit Alcohol Intake
7. Maintain a Healthy Weight
8. Manage Cholesterol Levels
9. Treat Atrial Fibrillation (AFib)
10. Regular Health Check-ups

Stroke prevention is about making informed lifestyle choices and managing health conditions effectively. By focusing on the above, individuals can significantly reduce their risk of stroke.

Stroke education and awareness play critical roles in recognising the symptoms (F.A.S.T) and understanding the importance of prevention.

Always consult with a healthcare provider for personalised advice and strategies tailored to individual health needs.

Secondary Stroke Prevention

Secondary stroke, refers to someone who has already survived a previous stroke or TIA.

Preventing a secondary stroke requires some drastic changes in lifestyle and eating habits. This may involve being placed on numerous medications to control hypertension, cholesterol, diabetes, and/or blood thinners. A change in diet and regular exercise is essential. Smoking should be strongly discouraged, and smokers need to quit as soon as possible.

Stress, often referred to as the silent killer, should be managed carefully. Stroke survivors already face significant stress as they adjust to their new realities, and the initial shock of experiencing a stroke can be overwhelming in itself.

Early Warning Signs - F.A.S.T

Stroke early warning signs are easily recognisable when using the acronym F.A.S.T.. If you suspect a stroke, perform an assessment, and if ANY of the following signs are present, seek immediate medical help, as the person could be experiencing a life-threatening stroke. Time is of the essence as brain cells will be dying. Wasted time means wasted brain cells.

F - is for face; look for any drooping on one side of the face?

A - is for arms; is the individual able to raise both arms equally and hold them there?

S - is for speech; are they able to speak clearly or are they slurring their words?

T - is for time; time is of the essence, call the emergency services and seek immediate medical help.

Performing the F.A.S.T. assessment could save someone's life.

Remember F.A.S.T. saves lives

The New Normal

What is normal?

"Normal" describes a condition, state, or behaviour that is considered typical or standard within a specific context. It often represents what is regarded as usual or average, whether relating to physical health, social behaviour, or other aspects of life.

Defining normal is complex; what might be normal for one person may seem abnormal to another.

Enduring a stroke that results in permanent or partial paralysis is not only a devastating experience for the survivor. It has far-reaching effects on everyone around them. The world they once knew has abruptly changed. The "normal" life they once experienced has taken on a completely new meaning. Although surviving such a terrifying ordeal brings relief and joy to the survivor's family, the reality that follows can be challenging.

Keep in mind that the survivor may no longer be able to tackle tasks as easily as they once did. It's as if a tornado has swept through their mind, leaving a trail of overwhelming and irreversible damage in its wake of destruction.

The stroke has created a new reality that requires the survivor to adapt to a 'new normal' lifestyle. Without an instruction manual to guide them, survivors and caregivers do not know what to expect.

For starters, a survivor needs to recognise that what they had before the stroke may be gone. Now is the time to re-evaluate the situation, taking stock of what has been lost and what remains. By identifying what remains, you uncover the foundation for rebuilding. Focus all your attention on these strengths and progressively, through intensive therapy, begin rebuilding from there. Avoid dwelling on what has been lost; instead, look forward to what can be regained.

Emotional Liability

Nothing can prepare a caregiver and their family for the complex surge of emotions the survivor is about to experience. Having survived such an ordeal, they may look the same, but emotionally they are a train wreck, and may seam like a complete stranger. Initially, the overwhelming shock of what happened might make it difficult for them to manage their emotions. The first six months are often the hardest, but as they come to terms with what happened, things will gradually begin to improve.

Remember that they have endured a life-altering ordeal. The stroke has caused brain cell loss, resulting in damage that can lead to changes in behaviour. Occasional outbursts of profanity or slander may seem out of character compared to how you remember them. These reactions are symptoms of the stroke, not a reflection of who they are as a person. Don't hesitate to seek professional guidance from a Neuropsychologist

Survivors are prone to strong, uncontrollable emotions and sudden mood swings, a condition referred to as emotional liability. This emotional liability may be out of sync with their current environment and could lead to the Pseudobulbar Affect (PBA).

Pseudobulbar Affect (PBA)

The overwhelming emotional strain that is steadily accumulating could potentially trigger the Pseudobulbar Affect (PBA), a neurological condition characterised by sudden and uncontrollable episodes of laughter or crying, without any clear external cause.

PBA often manifests as inappropriate emotional responses that are out of sync with the surrounding context. For instance, a person with PBA might find themselves laughing uncontrollably during a solemn or tragic moment, or crying unexpectedly in response to something happy or joyful.

These outbursts can be confusing and distressing, both for the individual experiencing them and for those around them.

Pain

Stroke survivors often face the challenge of chronic post-stroke pain (It's like "pain on steroids"), which can develop immediately after the stroke or gradually over the following months.

This pain can manifest in many ways, often linked to nerve damage sustained during the stroke. The result is excruciating, persistent pain that can be difficult to describe in words. It's a type of pain that goes beyond anything most people can imagine and, for survivors, it can be relentless, affecting them 24/7.

A significant percentage of stroke survivors may develop Central Post-Stroke Pain (CPSP). A condition commonly characterised by a throbbing, shooting pain through the areas affected by the stroke. Some individuals may experience sensations such as pins and needles or numbness in these areas.

When asked to explain the pain the author experienced after his stroke, he struggled to find an adequate comparison. The closest analogy he could come up with was the pain of slamming a car door on his hand and then multiplying that pain tenfold. That might give you — the caregiver —a faint idea of the constant, all-encompassing pain that persisted every single day, around the clock

Hypersensitivity

After a stroke, the body becomes hypersensitive to stimuli like temperature and touch. Cold sensations may begin to feel hot, and any contact with the skin on the affected side can trigger a painful, burning sensation. Similarly, hot sensations may feel cold. In such cases, the person may not be aware that they are touching a heat source and could burn themselves without knowing or feeling it.

Sitting on a leather or plastic-covered couch may cause the skin to sweat, leading to the skin sticking to the material. When trying to move off the couch, this can create a painful sensation, making the survivor feel as though their skin is slowly being peeled away from their body.

It's important to show empathy for their complaints. This isn't an act or a plea for attention— the pain they experience is very real.

Fatigue After Stroke

One of the biggest misconceptions about stroke survivors is that they are lazy. In reality, they are anything but that. Stroke survivors have suffered damage to the brain, and this means they must work four times harder than most individuals to accomplish what others may take for granted. The effort required to complete even simple tasks can exhaust even the most resilient survivor, forcing them to rest.

As a caregiver, it's important to approach the situation with empathy, always keeping in mind the challenges the survivor is facing. They have no control over how quickly they tire. The brain is tirelessly working to repair damaged pathways, so it needs all the rest it can get.

When a survivor frequently complains of pain and fatigue, listen carefully. Brain damage is an invisible injury that can result in severe pain and exhaustion.

The survivor is not exaggerating; the discomfort that they're experiencing is very real.

Home Modifications

When homes are initially designed, they often overlook the needs of individuals with disabilities, making modifications necessary for survivors. These changes will vary for each individual, tailored to accommodate their specific needs while ensuring their safety.

One of the most hazardous areas in the home is the bathroom. With its sharp corners, hard surfaces, and slippery floors, it's crucial to install grab rails—at least inside the shower, near the toilet, and in any other areas deemed necessary for support.

Additionally, a plastic, non-slip shower chair and a hand-held shower-head are essential for the survivor to bathe safely. Clear a space around the toilet to allow wheelchair access for safe and easy transfers.

Furniture, ornaments, large plants, and loose rugs should be relocated or stored away to allow easy wheelchair access. Those loose rugs and mats will create dangerous obstacles for wheelchairs and for the survivor, especially when they start learning to walk. Any unnecessary obstacles will increase the risk of falls.

If your home has stairs, consider adding a ramp for wheelchair accessibility. Before installing any permanent modifications, ensure the ramp's angle is safe and accessible. Safety should always be the top priority when making any modifications.

In the kitchen, reposition crockery and utensils to more accessible locations. You may also need to clear certain areas to allow safe movement for wheelchair access.

Frustration vs Anger

The sudden loss of abilities can lead to frustrating situations, prompting lifestyle changes that are difficult to adapt to. From the outside, these frustrations may sometimes appear as angry outbursts. If you're unfamiliar with what they're going through, it's easy to misinterpret frustration as anger. Before reacting or making quick judgments, try to put yourself in their shoes and view things from their perspective. For example, a simple task like opening a coffee jar can be incredibly frustrating when you can only use one hand.

To gain a better understanding of their daily struggles, try tying one hand behind your back and going about your day. You may be surprised by just how challenging even the most simple of tasks becomes, which will give you an insight into their daily experiences. Be observant, and try to recognise and anticipate situations that might be frustrating for them. Whenever possible, offer help or, even better, rearrange items to make them more accessible. Allowing them to attempt tasks independently— under supervision of course —can help retrain their brain and restore some confidence.

Rehabilitation is a long and difficult journey. Doing everything for them may foster dependence, hindering their progress. Patience is crucial—responding to their frustrations with anger will only escalate the situation. Instead, take a deep breath, remain calm, and support them as they move forward.

Stress and Recovery

Stroke recovery is a particularly challenging chapter in a survivor's life. The journey back to health is often slow and gradual, requiring patience and resilience. Minimising additional stress during this time is essential, as extra pressure or anxiety can hinder recovery and heighten the risk of further complications, including an unwelcome secondary stroke.

By creating a calm, supportive environment, you help lay the foundation for steady progress, giving the survivor the best chance to heal and rebuild their life.

Loneliness

Adversity often reveals who your true friends are, with misunderstanding and discomfort often causing some people to drift away. Many simply don't know how to act or what to say during difficult times, and human nature often leads them to avoid uncomfortable situations. Unfortunately, this avoidance isn't limited to friends—family members may also fall into this pattern, unintentionally isolating the survivor.

Separated from friends and family, the survivor may quickly slip into loneliness, which, if unaddressed, can intensify feelings of isolation and lead to depression.

Depression

Experiencing depression after a stroke is not only common but also often recognisable. Changes in mood and a loss of interest in previously enjoyable activities are typical signs of this condition. Apathy may arise due to the trauma the brain endures during a stroke. Thankfully, modern medicine offers effective treatments to help manage depression, so survivors don't have to feel this way. Seeking medical assistance without delay is essential.

If there are any thoughts of suicide, it is crucial to take them seriously and seek immediate professional help. The sudden loss of independence can leave a survivor feeling hopeless, potentially leading to an increased reliance on others. They may even start to believe that the world would be better off without them, and such distressing thoughts must be addressed and never ignored.

If left unaddressed, these feelings can escalate into a more serious situation. It is essential for survivors to speak with a qualified professional who specialises in neuro-mental disorders—a neuropsychologist. This type of professional, detached from the situation and not personally involved, can provide objective support, guidance, and help them navigate this difficult time.

It's important to remember that, despite our expectations, we are all human and not always equipped to handle every challenge life presents. For family and friends who remain by the survivor's side, it is crucial to offer reassurance and express love and care.

Let the survivor know that their health and well-being are your top priorities, and provide as much emotional support as possible. Your encouragement can make a significant difference in their recovery journey.

Anxiety

When a stroke survivor first ventures out into public—whether it's a trip to the grocer's or for a cup of coffee—they may experience a wave of anxiety. Feelings of self-consciousness can be overwhelming, creating the impression that everyone is watching them. It's important to reassure them that this perception is unfounded.

To avoid these uncomfortable situations, some survivors may choose to stay isolated within the safety of their homes. It's common for people to be curious about someone with physical challenges, but they might not know the best way to approach the subject. Rather than feeling frustrated by their lack of understanding, try to use these moments as opportunities to educate others, helping them gain a better understanding of the situation.

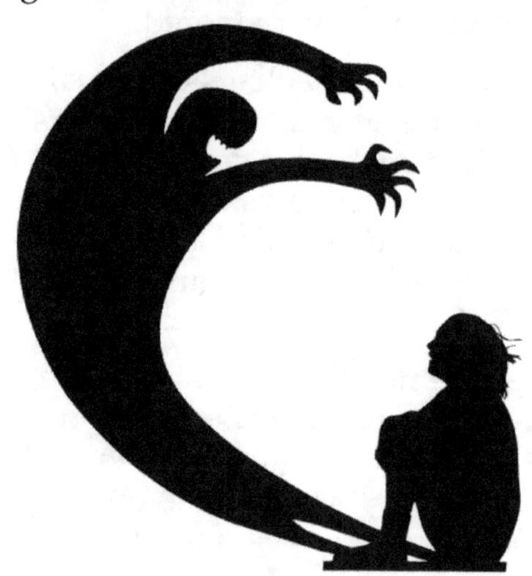

Remember, you have endured an experience that most people may never be exposed to and cannot fully comprehend. Rather than withdrawing, hold your head high and take pride in your journey as a survivor.

The encouraging news is that the more often you venture out into public, the more your anxiety will diminish. Start with small steps, gradually increasing your exposure to larger crowds. With each outing, you will gain confidence and become more at ease in public spaces, enabling you to eventually reclaim your place in society and embrace new experiences.

Dressing and Grooming

Getting dressed and grooming oneself are essential daily activities, but they can become significantly more difficult after a stroke, especially when using only one hand. Fortunately, having a caregiver to assist can greatly simplify these tasks.

Whether or not you have help, it is important to always lead with your weaker side. For example, when putting on a shirt, start by inserting your weak arm into the sleeve first, then follow with your stronger arm. The same approach applies when putting on trousers. Lead with the weak leg.

When it comes to shoes, assistance may be necessary initially, especially until you regain enough strength in your leg muscles to lift your foot comfortably. At first, opting for shoes with Velcro straps or no-tie shoelaces can make things much easier. While it is possible to tie shoelaces with one hand, it can be quite challenging.

Grooming can also be a hurdle, particularly if Hyper-sexuality dominant side was affected. However, with practice and patience, it will become easier over time. It's essential for survivors to avoid using razors or sharp objects on their own during this phase to ensure safety.

As you navigate these daily tasks, remember that progress takes time, and it is perfectly okay to ask for help when needed. With determination, the right attitude, and effective strategies, survivors can regain their independence in grooming and dressing.

Sex After a Stroke

While changes in sexual behaviour are not experienced by all stroke survivors, those who do may find it to be a sensitive topic and might avoid discussing it. These changes can include diminished libido, heightened sexual urges, impulsivity, or shifts in sexual preferences and behaviours.

Hyper-sexuality, or a heightened sexual desire following a stroke, is not typically observed. But if regions of the brain that control behaviour and impulse regulation —such as the frontal lobe, temporal lobe, or hypothalamus —are damaged, it might result in heightened sexual desires. In cases like this, it is crucial to seek medical advice, as there are ways of treating the condition.

What is more common, however, is for survivors to face difficulties such as diminished libido or challenges linked to paralysis, fatigue, or other physical limitations.

Under these circumstances, intimacy may still be possible. However, you should consult your doctor before engaging in any sexual activity to ensure that it is safe for you to do so.

Many survivors and their partners find that post stroke sex can still be just as enjoyable as it was before the stroke. While they may find certain sexual positions to be more challenging due to physical limitations, intimacy does not have to be limited to penetration alone. With a bit of creativity, foreplay can be just as exciting and fulfilling.

Intimacy encompasses much more than intercourse. It may be helpful to begin with activities such as kissing, caressing, or massaging, allowing both partners to reconnect emotionally and physically. It is important to take things slowly and openly communicate your feelings, concerns, and anxieties with your partner. This openness will help both of you explore and discover positions or techniques that feel comfortable and satisfying for both.

Patience and understanding are key to rekindling intimacy. By working together, experimenting with different approaches, and being mindful of each other's needs, you can create a fulfilling sexual experience that respects your individual limits and strengthens your bond.

Buffer Zone

In times of uncertainty and worry, it's completely understandable for friends and family to reach out for updates on the survivor's condition. They may call or ask for news through social media to stay informed about how things are progressing. During this period, it can be helpful for a family member or close friend to take on the role of a middleman, serving as a buffer between the survivor and the outside world.

This person can help manage communication, allowing the survivor to focus on their recovery without being overwhelmed by constant inquiries. By doing this, they can create a peaceful and supportive environment around the survivor, ensuring that they have the emotional space needed to heal.

It's important for the survivor to feel secure and cared for, and having someone dedicated to providing updates can alleviate some of the stress that comes from frequent questions and concerns. This approach not only protects the survivor's well-being but also helps keep friends and family connected without adding unnecessary pressure.

Medication and Side Effects

After a stroke, survivors often find themselves on a new regimen of medications, which can be more than they're used to. Many of these medications come with a range of side effects, some of which can be quite daunting. Unfortunately, it's not uncommon for the family of the survivor to struggle to get the medical staff to take their concerns seriously.

Family members and caregivers should make it a priority to become familiar with all the medications prescribed, including their potential side effects. Being informed is crucial, as it enables them to recognise when the survivor begins to behave differently due to the medication. If such changes occur, it's essential to seek medical help right away and inform the healthcare team about what's happening.

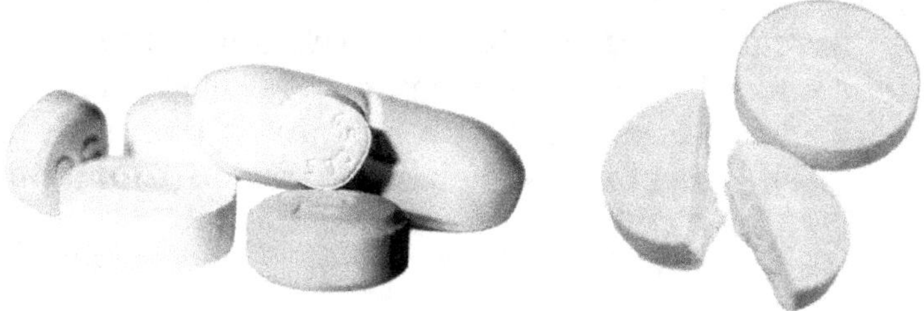

Remember, you are the survivor's advocate. Don't hesitate to hold the doctor accountable until all your questions are answered and you receive clear solutions. The best way to approach this is by asking plenty of questions. For example, you can ask, "What can we do about this side effect?" or "Is there an alternative medication that might work better?"

Being proactive and engaged in their care is key to ensuring the best possible outcomes.

Neuroplasticity

The survivor's family may encounter an indifferent attitude from the medical staff, who mistakenly believe that survivors only have two years to regain as much mobility as possible, after which no further progress can be made.

It is this dismissive attitude that may cause survivors and their family's to lose hope after such a short period of time. This outdated belief no longer holds true.

It has been discovered that the brain, with its neuroplasticity, continues to learn and adapt throughout an individual's lifetime. "Neuro" refers to the brain, while "plasticity" refers to its flexibility. Therefore, neuroplasticity is the brain's ability to reorganise itself by forming new neural connections throughout the life of the individual. It turns out that the brain begins learning the day we are born and ceases the day we die.

With the brain constantly working to repair itself, it makes recovery possible many years after the initial trauma.

A Positive Attitude Yields Positive Results

Don't expect everything to be fine right away. Recovery is a deliberate process that requires arduous hours of repetition. Patience and perseverance are the keys to a productive rehabilitation. Motivating the survivor as much as possible will get them moving, but it is their determination to get better that will keep them going. Don't ever give up.

Technology is advancing at such a rampant pace and scientists are continually finding new ways to help survivors recover from their harrowing ordeal.

Even the toughest of the tough, the "well-adjusted" survivor who thinks they are doing well, are going to have some tough days. Delayed reactions are par to recovery.

Many survivors steel themselves to their loss and feel strong. That is, until the first sign of hope, whether it's a finger twitch or standing for the first time. The slightest whisper of hope will cause a seasoned survivor's eyes to well-up with tears of joy. That twitch of hope is enough to instil confidence. Hang in there, for as long as it takes.

As a caregiver, re-enforce how proud you are of them – over and over again, session after session, year after year. Never give up hope. The more love and affection they encounter, the more determined they will be to recover! Recovery is a slooooooooow and tedious process —I am talking glacial speed— don't expect overnight miracles. Every action begins with the tiniest of twitches. The recovery process may slow down, but it will only stop when you, and only you, decide to give up.

Never give up and remember that *no is never an option.*

Caregiver

In the blink of an eye, a loved one can become a caregiver. Changing their life forever —and forever is a long time.

Research indicates that many informal caregivers are unprepared for the demands of this role, and provide care without adequate support. Over one-third of caregivers who continue offering intensive care end up compromising their own health.

Caregiving is a 24/7 responsibility, potentially one of the most demanding and challenging tasks you'll ever face, with little to no recognition or reward. Survivors of brain injuries might struggle with emotional control, leading to frustration as they struggle to perform everyday tasks they once managed easily. This emotional frustration can manifest in ways that seem harsh or abrupt, now that they lack the emotional intelligence to express themselves in a more controlled manner, which can be disheartening.

In that same instant, a breadwinner can become unemployable, passing the financial burden onto others. With a long and slow recovery process, medical bills can quickly accumulate, creating a financial situation that the caregiving partner can ill afford.

Without a steady income, a stay-at-home informal caregiver will see their savings dwindling into a medical black hole. As dire as it may be, returning to work is not always an option as it would require the hiring a full-time caregiver, a situation that many cannot afford. Caught between a rock and a hard place, informal caregivers may find themselves juggling many balls at once. Sharing the caregiving responsibilities is essential.

It is important for informal caregivers to prioritise their own well-being, carving out time in their busy day to recharge in a way that helps them cope during challenging times. Recognising when to seek help—even if just for a short period—is crucial.

A caregiver who is mentally and physically drained cannot effectively care for anyone, including themselves.

As a caregiver, you are expected to be a pillar of support throughout this difficult journey, often going beyond simply offering love and reassurance.

It is also your responsibility to raise concerns about any unnecessary risks that may endanger their life or safety.

Therapy

A crucial component of the stroke rehabilitation process.

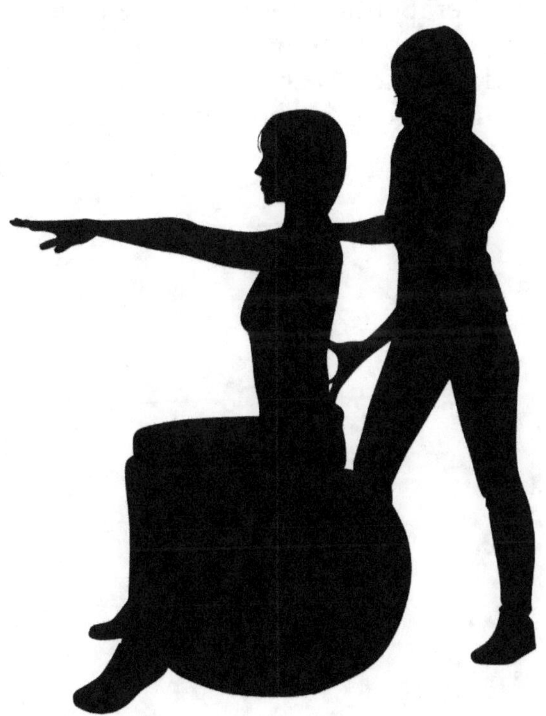

Physiotherapy

Physical therapy, often referred to as physiotherapy or simply PT, is a type of rehabilitation that involves physical treatments aimed at restoring movement and functionality to injured areas of the body. The primary goal of physical therapy is to help individuals improve their quality of life through enhanced mobility.

For stroke survivors, physiotherapy plays a crucial role in recovery, particularly focusing on the lower limbs. The therapy is designed to help regain balance and improve walking ability, which are essential for overall independence.

Notably, the lower limbs tend to be the first part of the body to respond to therapeutic interventions, making them a key focus during rehabilitation. By engaging in targeted exercises and physical activities, stroke survivors can gradually rebuild strength, coordination, and confidence in their mobility.

Occupational Therapy

Occupational Therapy (OT) specialises in helping individuals regain and maintain the use of their upper limbs—the shoulder, arm, and hand. Occupational therapists work to enhance the skills necessary for daily living and work activities, tailoring their approach to the specific needs of each patient.

They assist people with physical, mental, or cognitive challenges, striving to restore independence by identifying and removing barriers in the environment. The role of an occupational therapist centres on improving participation in everyday tasks and enhancing overall functioning.

They achieve this by adapting the environment and modifying tasks to align with the individual's abilities. This may involve teaching essential skills not only to the patient but also to their family members, creating a supportive network for ongoing recovery and independence. Through personalised strategies and interventions, occupational therapists empower individuals to fully engage in their daily lives.

Speech Therapy

Speech therapists, also known as speech-language pathologists, specialise in assessing and treating a wide range of communication issues, including difficulties with voice and speech. Beyond enhancing communication skills, these professionals also address swallowing disorders, which can profoundly impact a person's quality of life.

Their expertise encompasses working with individuals who have difficulty speaking clearly, understanding language, or using their voice effectively. They also provide support for those with swallowing difficulties, known as dysphagia.

Treatment often involves creating personalised exercises, strategies, and techniques to improve communication skills and promote safe swallowing practices. By addressing both communication and swallowing challenges, speech therapists play a crucial role in helping individuals post-stroke regain confidence and independence in daily activities.

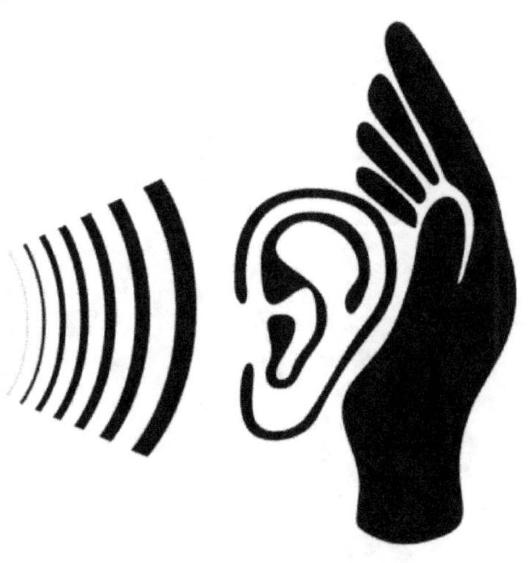

Psychologist

A psychologist is a professional that is detached from a situation, and who can approach it with a clear and open mind.

Following a stroke it is important for a survivor and caregiver to seek out a Neuropsychologist.

Is there a difference between a Psychologist and a Neuropsychologist, you may ask?

Yes, a psychologist is a mental health professional who studies and treats emotional, mental, and behavioural disorders where as a Neuropsychologist is a specialised psychologist who focuses on the relationship between the brain and behaviour.

A neuropsychologist specialises in helping individuals who have experienced brain injuries, neurological disorders, or cognitive impairments. They focus on assessing how these conditions affect cognitive functions, such as memory, attention, and problem-solving abilities.

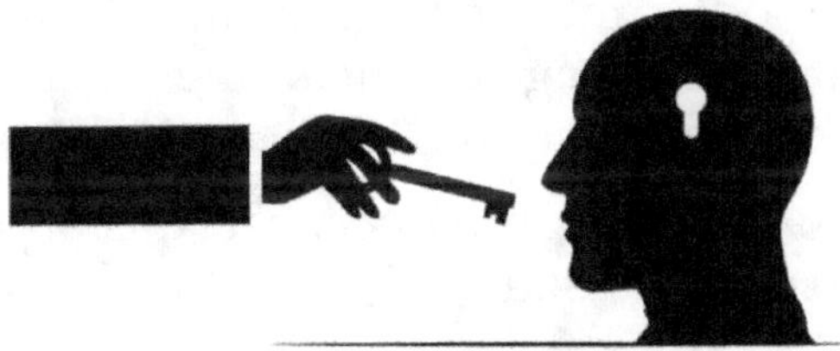

By conducting thorough evaluations, neuropsychologists can identify whether changes in a person's cognitive abilities or emotional behaviours are linked to their brain injury. This understanding allows them to create targeted treatment plans that address both cognitive and emotional challenges, ultimately helping patients improve their quality of life and regain independence.

5 Stages of Grief

A positive mindset is vital for a productive recovery, along with countless hours of repetitive therapy.

Stroke is a family affliction that affects not only the survivor but also their loved ones. It signifies the harsh reality of the "death" of the person they once knew and loved so dearly, along with the rebirth of a "new" survivor in their place. It is essential to learn to accept the survivor as they are. Their change in behaviour can be extremely challenging and emotional for everyone close to them.

A grieving period is therefore necessary, to navigate the various emotional stages, including denial, anger, bargaining, depression, and finally acceptance.

These steps do not necessarily occur in this order and can vary from person to person

Denial

Denial is not a river in Africa. It is real and can leave a person feeling numb, disoriented, and overwhelmed by the events that have just unfolded.

It's a natural reaction which passes with time.

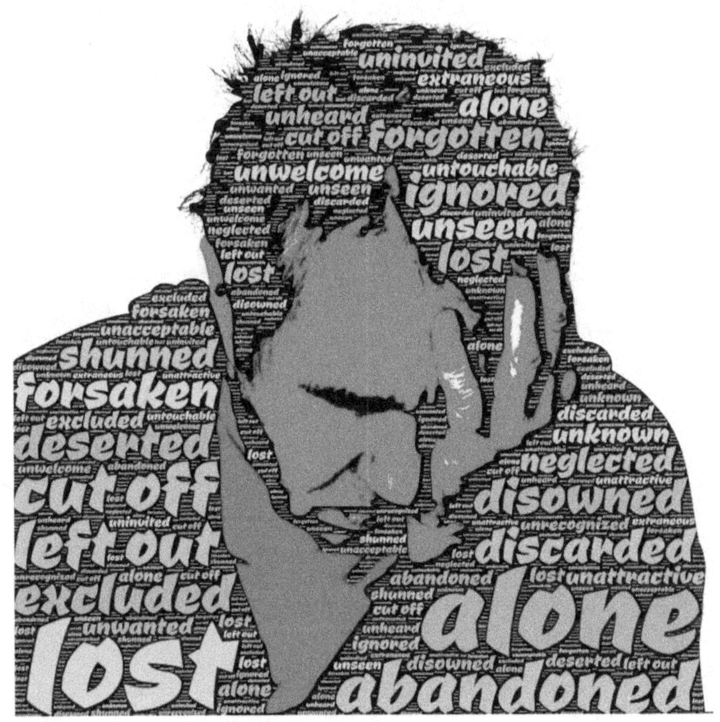

Anger

Anger is a common occurrence among stroke survivors.

They may find themselves frustrated and unsettled, caught in a chaotic whirlwind as they grapple with the drastic changes to their lifestyle. This sudden and unexpected shift can lead to outbursts of anger, which might be directed at anyone in close proximity be it friends, family, or caregivers—anyone whom they feel they can blame for their situation.

The abrupt loss of independence is devastating, and coming to terms with their deficits can be equally overwhelming.

Bargaining or negotiating

Bargaining or negotiating is when they find themselves asking many questions.

Questions such as: 'What if I had only' and wondering what they could have done differently, 'If only I could have one more chance' or 'If only I had done..... differently.'

Attempting to negotiate with their loss is an all too familiar scenario. Coming to terms with what has just happened to them, is tough.

Depression

Depression is the most easily recognisable sign and commonly expected with such a loss.

Regrettably, it does not only affect the survivor, instead, it touches all who are close to them. Each person may be affected to a different degree. Those not directly affected may not realise the impact it has on the family and what they are going through. They might even expect them to snap out of this stage of depression and sadness and to get on with their lives, which is easier said than done.

The family have just 'lost' a loved one, someone they love so dearly. They need to mourn their loss and accept the new survivor that has emerged in their place. Life for them has just taken a drastic turn and their future is now filled with ambiguity and vagueness.

No one can handle such adversity on their own and will need to seek out professional help, someone they can talk freely to about what they are going through. Professional help, preferably with a Neuropsychologist, is highly recommended for anyone close to the survivor.

A Neuropsychologist is someone who specialises in brain trauma and who is detached from the situation and trained to assist in such trying times.

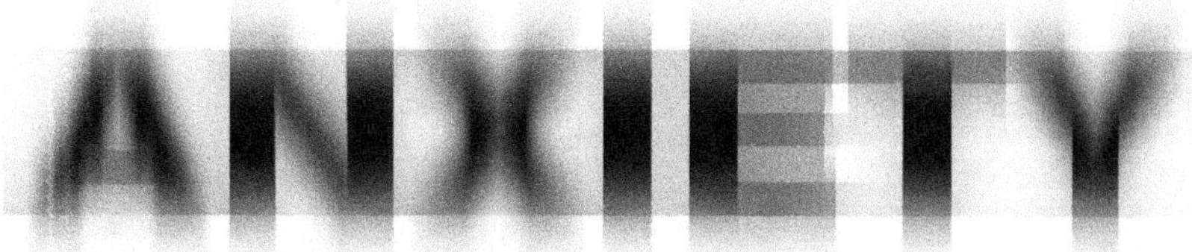

Having been through such a traumatic experience, nothing can prepare you for the tsunami of emotional upsurges that you are about to encounter.

With the road ahead filled with so much ambiguity, you need the assistance of someone with a clear head. Someone you can talk to, who can guide you through this upsurge.

Acceptance

Coming to terms with the reality of being a stroke survivor is one of the hardest stages to acknowledge.

Accepting a future filled with deficits and uncertainties is no easy task, and coming to terms with the possibility of relying on others for basic daily tasks can be equally challenging. Acceptance represents the stage at which they finally acknowledge what has happened. It is the point where they make peace with their new reality and prepare to begin the demanding journey of recovery.

Reaching acceptance does not mean giving up hope; rather, it marks the moment when they are ready to focus on adapting to their situation and rebuilding their independence. This stage is essential, as it allows them to engage fully with the rehabilitation process, facing each step with resilience and determination.

Empathy

Chores that were once taken for granted, tasks that could be done with eyes shut, may suddenly become daunting undertakings requiring the assistance of a caregiver. Activities such as dressing or cooking, might necessitate assistance. Getting around might require the services of a driver. Personal hygiene could also require support.

Try to understand what the survivor is experiencing. They may feel powerless, resembling a child trapped in an adult's body. They might need help bathing or even washing after using the toilet. If you, as a caregiver, find this situation humiliating, consider the humiliation they are enduring. They never asked to be placed in such a predicament; a stroke has led them to this situation.

The survivor is now faced with many uncertainties they were never prepared for, be they physical or cognitive. You may find them asking numerous questions. Remember this, there are no stupid questions, you are dealing with a loved one who survived a brain trauma.

If the survivor is dealing with aphasia, they might become further frustrated and annoyed by their inability to communicate. In such cases, it is important to speak with medical staff about effective ways to communicate with your loved one.

Don't feel intimidated by the many questions they may pose—no one expects you to be a medical expert with all the answers. You are there to serve as a sounding board, someone who will listen without judgment. Allow them to express their thoughts and fears. Remember to remain positive and reassure them that you will support them one hundred percent of the way. Listen to their fears and emotional anxieties; after all, they have been through a traumatic experience.

Keep offering as much emotional reassurance as you can.

Hyperbaric Oxygen Therapy (HBOT)

Hyperbaric Oxygen Therapy (HBOT) is a medical treatment used to enhance the body's natural healing processes by increasing the amount of oxygen delivered to tissues, especially for patients recovering from Brain Injuries.

What is Hyperbaric Oxygen Therapy?

Before getting started, we need to first understand the meaning of Hyperbaric. 'Hyperbaric' is an operating pressure that is greater than normal atmospheric pressure. Therefore, HBOT is the administering of oxygen under increased pressure.

Hyperbaric Oxygen Therapy (HBOT) is a medical treatment in which a patient is enclosed in a full-body chamber and exposed to high levels of oxygen at pressures greater than atmospheric pressure.

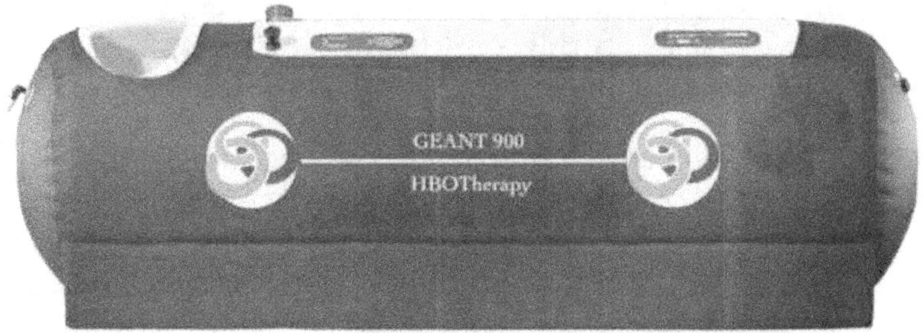

Under normal circumstances at sea level, a column of air with a pressure of one atmosphere (ATA) is exerted on the body.

As we ascend in altitude, the pressure decreases, increasing the size of the gas molecules in the column of air. On the other hand, when we descend, the reverse happens and the pressure increases, reducing the size of the individual gas molecules.

How Does It Work?

Hyperbaric Oxygen Therapy (HBOT) works by increasing the pressure in a controlled environment in an enclosed chamber and delivering larger amounts of oxygen to the patient.

HBOT is Based on Two Laws:

- **Henrys Law** which states that "At a constant temperature, the amount of a given gas that dissolves in a given type and volume of liquid is directly proportional to the partial pressure of that gas in equilibrium with that liquid. In other words, at a constant temperature, as the pressure increases on a liquid, so the liquid will be able to hold more gas molecules.

- **Dalton's Law** of Partial Pressure, states "that in a mixture of non-reacting gases, the total pressure exerted is equal to the sum of the partial pressures of the individual gases". In other words, the total pressure is made up of the sum of all the individual gases under pressure.

  i.e.: $P_{Total} = P_1 + P_2 + \ldots\ldots\ldots\ldots + P_n.$

This theory can easily be seen in everyday use, i.e. in soda drinks.

- **SODA EFFECT**: Soda is essentially syrup and water. Under normal conditions (one ATA), the pressure on the liquid is in equilibrium with the atmospheric pressure. By increasing the pressure in an enclosed container, we are able to dissolve carbon dioxide into the liquid and keep it there, whilst under pressure. Once the container is opened, the pressure is suddenly released and the CO_2 will come out of suspension and attempt to reach equilibrium, with the outside atmospheric pressure. This gives us the fizziness we all enjoy in our Sodas.

Once equilibrium is reached, we then refer to the soda as being flat.

Red blood cells have a limited capacity for binding oxygen to haemoglobin, the oxygen-carrying protein within these cells.

Blood plasma—the clear, yellowish fluid component of blood—carries approximately 3% of the body's oxygen concentration.

However, placing a patient in a hyperbaric environment with pressures greater than normal atmospheric levels, combined with elevated partial oxygen pressure, enables the body to dissolve more oxygen directly into red blood cells, plasma, cerebrospinal fluid, bone, and other bodily fluids.

This oxygen-saturated tissue can then reach all cells, tissues, and fluids in the body at higher-than-usual concentrations, significantly accelerating the body's natural healing processes.

Additionally, the elevated atmospheric pressure and oxygen levels help reduce inflammation and stimulate the growth of new blood vessels into affected areas. By delivering oxygen to damaged tissues, the therapy supports the body's healing mechanisms, even when blood flow is compromised. Oxygen can still reach damaged tissues through plasma and surrounding bodily fluids, through a process known to as the doughnut affect.

Hyperbaric Oxygen Therapy is particularly beneficial for treating wounds with limited blood flow or injuries where tissue swelling is present. Daily exposure to higher oxygen levels aids the body in expediting wound healing and overall recovery.

What Pressure is used?

Portable hyperbaric chambers are typically pressurised to 1.3 ATA, about 0.3 ATA above the ambient atmospheric pressure—roughly equivalent to the pressure felt at the bottom of a swimming pool's deep end.

The heightened oxygen concentration boosts the effectiveness of white blood cells— the essential components of the immune system that defend the body against infections and harmful agents — enhancing the body's self-healing capabilities.

Does it hurt?

Hyperbaric Oxygen Therapy is a painless, non-evasive procedure.

What to expect

When the chamber begins pressurising, patients may feel a change in pressure in their ears, similar to the sensation experienced when an aeroplane descends.

Swallowing or yawning can usually relieve any discomfort; alternatively, the Valsalva manoeuvre will help.

The Valsalva manoeuvre is achieved by closing your mouth and pinching your nose shut. Gently blow against the pinched nose. This will force air through the Eustachian tube and sinuses, equalising the pressure between the inner ear and the chamber's ambient pressure. Once the pressure is equalised, you can stop pinching your nose shut and gently blowing.

The ears will remain in equilibrium at a constant pressure. If the pressure increases you may have to repeat the procedure. At the end of each session, as the chamber pressure is reduced back to atmospheric levels, you don't have to do anything as the ears will naturally equalise themselves.

The "Doughnut Effect

Injured tissue forms a pattern resembling a doughnut. The centre, or "hole," represents the traumatised area—damaged tissue that has been directly impacted, such as the dead tissue following a stroke. Unfortunately, this central tissue cannot be revived. However, surrounding the dead core is inflamed dormant, yet still viable, tissue that forms a "doughnut" ring around the trauma. This tissue is compromised, limiting blood flow and oxygen delivery due to the inflammation.

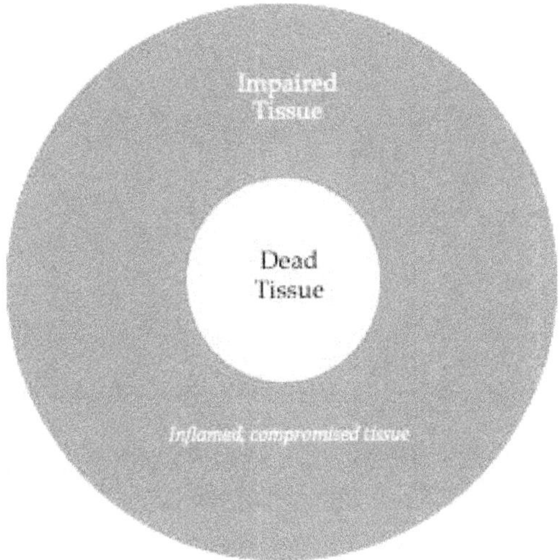

Placing a patient in a hyperbaric chamber and administering oxygen under pressure allows oxygen molecules to reduce in size, enabling them to penetrate the compromised tissue.

The combination of the hyperbaric environment and the higher partial pressure of oxygen promotes greater oxygen saturation into blood cells, plasma, cerebrospinal fluid, bone, and other bodily fluids. This increased oxygen concentration enhances white blood cell activity, stimulating the immune system, which supports the body's innate healing process.

Under these conditions, oxygen can now reach the inflamed dormant tissue in increased concentrations. The additional oxygen absorbed encourages new blood vessel growth within the affected area, helping to alleviate inflammation. By boosting oxygen levels in damaged tissues, the body's natural healing mechanisms can function more effectively, even when blood supply is restricted.

Through the diffusion of oxygen via plasma and other body fluids, damaged tissues initiate the repair process and promote recovery.

Electrical Stimulation

Electrical stimulation involves the use of electrical currents to stimulate nerves and muscles in patients recovering from stroke.

This therapeutic technique aims to improve motor function, enhance muscle strength, and promote neuroplasticity—the brain's ability to reorganise itself by forming new neural connections.

Electrical Muscle Stimulation (EMS)

Electrical Muscle Stimulation (EMS) involves the use of electrical currents, generated by a battery-operated device, to stimulate muscles. The device connects to the skin through two or more strategically placed electrodes, each carrying either a positive or negative charge. As the current flows between these electrodes, it triggers muscle contractions, effectively stimulating the targeted muscles.

The device's intensity and duration of electrical current can be adjusted to suit different needs, and it can be programmed for various cycles to optimise muscle engagement and relaxation. EMS is commonly used in fitness, rehabilitation, and physical therapy to enhance muscle strength, improve endurance, and support recovery.

Transcutaneous Electrical Nerve Stimulation (TENS)

Transcutaneous Electrical Nerve Stimulation (TENS) is a therapeutic technique that uses electrical currents, generated by a small, battery-operated device, to stimulate nerves for pain relief. TENS units deliver specific types of electrical pulses through the skin to target underlying nerves, helping to alleviate discomfort in various parts of the body. These devices come with two or more electrodes that are carefully placed on the skin over the areas needing treatment. The electrodes deliver controlled currents, which interact with nerve pathways and can reduce the sensation of pain.

TENS therapy is widely recognised for its effectiveness in managing both acute and chronic pain, and its portability makes it a convenient, non-invasive pain management option.

Functional Electrical Stimulation (FES)

Functional Electrical Stimulation (FES) is a technology that uses electrical stimulation to help survivors perform everyday activities. The device connects to the skin through two strategically placed electrodes, one carrying a positive charge and the other a negative. As the current flows between these electrodes, it triggers the nerves and muscles, effectively stimulating the targeted area, initiating muscle contractions.

One of its most common applications is to assist individuals with dorsiflexion. A function crucial for safe walking and running, as it raises the front of the foot from the ankle to allow the leg to safely swing forward, thus preventing it from dragging on the ground. This smooth motion allows the foot to clear the floor below it to prevent tripping and ensures a steady, balanced stride.

Normally, we perform this movement unconsciously. However, when an injury or illness disrupts this process, it requires conscious effort with each step to avoid falling, highlighting the importance of dorsiflexion for smooth movement.

Damage to the brain, nerves, or spinal cord can result in a condition known as "foot drop," in which the ability to lift the foot at the ankle is lost. This condition is often caused by damage to or loss of signals to the peroneal nerve, leading to the foot drooping and causing the toes to drag along the ground. Without dorsiflexion, walking becomes unstable, and the foot slaps down instead of rolling from heel to toe, increasing the risk of falls.

To avoid tripping, individuals with foot drop often compensate by swinging their leg in a circular motion, known as "circumduction." While this can help prevent stumbling, it puts strain on other joints and muscles, potentially leading to further complications.

Alternatively, people with foot drop may use an ankle-foot orthosis (AFO), a supportive brace that helps keep the foot raised. While effective, AFOs can be bulky and uncomfortable to wear for extended periods.

Recent advancements in FES technology offer a more comfortable and dynamic solution. Modern FES devices stimulate the necessary nerves and muscles to support a natural walking gait. These devices are synchronised with the user's walking pattern and use either a tilt sensor or a heel switch to activate the unit at the right time. The heel switch triggers when the heel of the foot leaves the ground, while the tilt switch activates when the leg tilts in preparation for the next step. In both cases, the device sends a small electrical pulse to the nerve, lifting the front of the foot from the ankle, allowing for a smoother and more natural walking motion.

Individuals using FES for foot drop experience improved stability, greater mobility, and a reduced risk of falls. FES helps them to regain confidence and independence in their daily activities.

295 stroke medical terms explained in layman's terms

Agnosia:

Difficulty recognising familiar objects or people.

Aneurysm Clipping:

A surgical procedure to treat a brain aneurysm.

Aneurysm Coiling:

A technique to block blood flow into an aneurysm.

Aneurysm:

A weak spot in a blood vessel that can balloon and burst.

Angiogenesis:

The formation of new blood vessels, important in stroke recovery.

Angiogram:

An imaging test using contrast dye to visualise blood vessels.

Angioplasty and Stent Placement:

Techniques to open narrowed blood vessels.

Angioplasty:

A procedure to open narrowed or blocked blood vessels.

Angiotensin-Converting Enzyme (ACE) Inhibitors:

Medications used to lower blood pressure.

Anhidrosis:

Reduced ability to sweat.

Anoxia:

Lack of oxygen, potentially damaging brain tissue.

Anticoagulant:

Medication to prevent blood clots.

Anticoagulation Clinic:

A specialised clinic that monitors patients on blood-thinning medications.

Anticoagulation Therapy:

Medication to prevent blood from clotting.

Anticonvulsant:

Medication to prevent seizures.

Antiemetic Medications:

Drugs used to control nausea and vomiting.

Antiemetic Patches:

Transdermal patches that release medication to prevent nausea and vomiting.

Antiemetic:

A medication to prevent or alleviate nausea and vomiting.

Antihypertensive Medications:

Drugs that lower high blood pressure.

Antiplatelet Medications:

Drugs that prevent platelets from sticking together.

Antipyretic Medications:

Drugs used to reduce fever.

Antispasmodic Medications:

Drugs that reduce muscle spasms.

Aphasia:

Difficulty speaking or understanding language after a stroke.

Aphaeresis:

A procedure to remove specific components from the blood, such as plasma or platelets.

Aphonia:

Loss of voice or inability to produce sound.

Apneustic:

Abnormal breathing characterised by prolonged pauses between breaths.

Apnoea:

Temporary cessation of breathing.

Apoplexy:

A term used in the past to describe a sudden stroke.

Arterial Blood Gas (ABG) Test:

A blood test to assess oxygen and carbon dioxide levels.

Arteriogram:

An X-ray test to visualise blood vessels.

Arteriosclerosis:

Hardening and narrowing of the arteries.

Arteriovenous (AV) Fistula:

An abnormal connection between an artery and a vein.

Arteriovenous Fistula (AVF):

An abnormal connection between an artery and a vein.

Arteriovenous Malformation (AVM):

Abnormal tangles of blood vessels in the brain.

Aspiration:

Inhaling foreign substances into the lungs, a risk in those with swallowing difficulties.

Asymmetric:

Not equal or balanced on both sides.

Asymptomatic:

Showing no symptoms or signs of illness.

Asystole:

The absence of any electrical activity in the heart, a medical emergency.

Ataxia:

Loss of coordination, often seen in stroke patients.

Ataxic Gait:

An unsteady and uncoordinated walking pattern.

Atrial Fibrillation (AFib):

An irregular heartbeat that increases stroke risk.

Atrophy:

The shrinking or wasting away of tissue, often seen in muscles after a stroke.

Autonomic Dysreflexia:

An exaggerated response to certain stimuli in individuals with spinal cord injuries.

Autonomic Nervous System:

The part of the nervous system controlling involuntary functions.

Axon:

The long, slender part of a nerve cell that transmits signals.

Bacteraemia:

Presence of bacteria in the bloodstream, potentially leading to infection.

Bilateral:

Affecting both sides of the body or brain.

Blood Thinners:

Medications to prevent blood clots.

Brachial Plexus:

A network of nerves in the shoulder region that controls arm movement.

Bradykinesia:

Slowness of movement, often seen in Parkinson's disease and some stroke cases.

Bradyphrenia:

Slowed thinking or cognitive processing.

Brain Bleed:

Bleeding inside the brain, which is common in haemorrhagic strokes.

Brain Infarction:

Tissue death in the brain caused by a lack of blood supply.

Cardiac Catheterisation:

A procedure to diagnose and treat heart conditions.

Cardiac Monitoring:

Continuous tracking of heart activity, crucial in stroke management.

Cardiologist:

A heart specialist who may be involved in stroke care.

Cardiopulmonary Resuscitation (CPR):

Emergency lifesaving measures for cardiac arrest.

Carotid Artery:

The main arteries in the neck that supply blood to the brain.

Carotid Dissection:

A tear in the carotid artery, which can lead to stroke.

Carotid Endarterectomy:

Surgical removal of plaque from the carotid arteries.

Carotid Stenosis:

Narrowing of the carotid arteries.

Catheter-Associated Urinary Tract Infection (CAUTI):

An infection related to urinary catheter use.

Catheter:

A thin tube used for various medical purposes.

Catheterisation:

Inserting a thin tube into a body cavity or blood vessel.

Cerebellum:

The part of the brain responsible for coordination and balance.

Cerebral Angioedema:

Swelling in the brain due to an allergic reaction or other causes.

Cerebral Angiography:

Imaging of blood vessels in the brain.

Cerebral Collateral Circulation:

Alternative blood pathways in the brain that can compensate for reduced flow.

Cerebral Edema:

Swelling of the brain due to fluid buildup.

Cerebral Hemodynamics:

Blood flow in the brain.

Cerebral Perfusion Pressure (CPP):

The pressure needed to maintain blood flow to the brain.

Cerebral Vasculitis:

Inflammation of blood vessels in the brain.

Cerebral Vasospasm:

Abnormal narrowing of cerebral blood vessels.

Cerebrospinal Angiography:

Imaging of blood vessels in the brain and spinal cord.

Cerebrospinal Fluid (CSF):

The fluid that surrounds the brain and spinal cord.

Cerebrovascular Accident (CVA):

A medical term for a stroke.

Cervical Discectomy:

Surgical removal of a cervical disc.

Cholecystectomy:

Surgical removal of the gallbladder.

Cholesterol Plaque:

Fatty deposits that can narrow blood vessels.

Clot Buster:

Medication that dissolves blood clots.

Coagulation:

The process of blood clotting.

Cognition:

Mental processes such as thinking, learning, and memory.

Collateral Circulation:

Extra blood vessels that can provide an alternative route for blood flow in case of a blockage. They act as backup pathways to nourish the brain and reduce the impact of a stroke.

Corticosteroids:

Medications used to reduce inflammation and swelling.

Cranial Nerves:

Nerves connected directly to the brain, controlling various functions.

CT Scan (Computed Tomography):

A type of X-ray that shows brain images.

Cyanosis:

Bluish discolouration of the skin, often due to reduced oxygen levels.

Decannulate:

To remove a tracheostomy tube.

Decannulation:

The process of removing a tracheostomy tube.

Decompressive Craniotomy:

A surgical procedure to remove part of the skull to reduce pressure on the brain.

Deep Brain Stimulation (DBS):

A surgical treatment for neurological conditions.

Deep Vein Thrombosis (DVT) Prophylaxis:

Measures to prevent blood clots in deep veins.

Deep Vein Thrombosis (DVT):

Blood clot in a deep vein, a potential stroke risk factor.

Dextrocardia:

A condition where the heart is located on the right side of the chest.

Diplopia:

Double vision, a visual impairment sometimes seen in stroke patients.

Dizziness:

A common symptom during or after a stroke.

Dopamine:

A neurotransmitter involved in mood, movement, and reward.

Doppler Ultrasound:

A test that uses sound waves to check blood flow in the arteries.

Dysarthria:

Difficulty with speech due to muscle weakness.

Dysarthrosis:

Difficulty forming words due to muscle weakness.

Dysdiadochokinesia:

Difficulty with rapid alternating movements, such as hand-clapping.

Dyskinesia:

Involuntary, often erratic, muscle movements.

Dysmetria:

Difficulty with judging distance or coordinating movements.

Dysphagia Diet:

A modified diet for individuals with swallowing difficulties.

Dysphagia:

Difficulty swallowing.

Dysphasia:

Difficulty with language or communication, often related to stroke.

Dysphasic:

Experiencing language difficulties, such as speaking or understanding.

Dysphonia:

Abnormal voice production or difficulty speaking.

Dysphonia:

Difficulty with voice production, often affecting speech after a stroke.

Dysuria:

Painful or difficult urination.

Echocardiogram:

An ultrasound of the heart to assess its function.

Echocardiogram:

An ultrasound of the heart to check for heart-related stroke causes.

Edema:

Swelling due to fluid buildup.

Edrophonium Test:

A diagnostic test for certain neuromuscular disorders.

Electrocardiogram (ECG or EKG):

A test to measure electrical activity in the heart.

Electroencephalogram (EEG):

A test to measure brain electrical activity.

Embolectomy:

Surgical removal of an embolus (clot) from a blood vessel.

Embolism:

A blood clot or debris that travels through the bloodstream

and can cause a blockage.

Endarterectomy:

Surgical removal of plaque from an artery, such as the carotid artery.

Endovascular Aneurysm Repair (EVAR):

A minimally invasive procedure to treat aortic aneurysms.

Endovascular Coiling:

A procedure to treat certain types of brain aneurysms.

Epidural Haematoma:

Bleeding between the skull and the protective covering of the brain.

Epidural:

Located just outside the protective covering of the spinal cord.

Episodic Ataxia:

Brief episodes of uncoordinated movement, sometimes seen in stroke patients.

External Ventricular Drain (EVD):

A device to drain cerebrospinal fluid from the brain.

Extracorporeal Life Support (ECLS):

A system that takes over the heart and lung functions temporarily.

Extracorporeal Membrane Oxygenation (ECMO):

A life-support system for severe respiratory or cardiac failure.

Extra-cranial:

Outside the skull.

Extrapyramidal:

Related to movement control outside the pyramidal system (voluntary motor pathways).

Facial Droop:

A sagging or uneven appearance of the face, often a sign of stroke.

Facial Paralysis:

Loss of movement or sensation in the face, often due to nerve damage.

Fasciculations:

Involuntary muscle twitches.

Feeding Tube:

A device used to provide nutrition directly to the stomach or intestines.

Flaccidity:

Loss of muscle tone and strength.

Flail Chest:

Multiple broken ribs resulting in unstable chest wall

movement.

Fluoroscopy:

A real-time X-ray imaging technique used in certain procedures.

Gag Reflex:

The natural protective reflex to prevent choking.

Gait Disturbance:

Difficulty walking or maintaining balance.

Gingivitis:

Inflammation of the gums.

Glasgow Coma Scale:

A scale used to assess a patient's level of consciousness after a stroke.

Glottal Closure:

The act of the vocal cords coming together during speech.

Glottis:

The part of the throat containing the vocal cords.

Haematocrit:

A measure of the proportion of blood that consists of red blood cells.

Haemorrhage:

Bleeding, which can occur inside the brain during a haemorrhagic stroke.

Haemorrhagic Stroke:

Bleeding in the brain due to a ruptured blood vessel.

Haemorrhagic Transformation:

Conversion of an ischemic stroke into a haemorrhagic stroke.

Haemorrhoidectomy:

Surgical removal of haemorrhoids.

Haematoma:

A collection of blood outside blood vessels, often seen in haemorrhagic strokes.

Hemianopia:

Partial loss of vision in one or both eyes.

Hemiparesis:

Weakness on one side of the body.

Hemiparetic Gait:

A walking pattern characterised by weakness on one side of the body.

Hemiplegia:

Paralysis on one side of the body.

Hemoperfusion:

A technique to remove toxins from the blood.

Home Health Care:

Medical care provided in a patient's home, often during stroke recovery.

Hyperextension:

Excessive backward bending of a joint.

Hyperkalaemia:

Elevated levels of potassium in the blood.

Hyperlipidaemia:

Elevated levels of fats (lipids) in the blood, which can contribute to stroke risk.

Hyperreflexia:

Exaggerated reflexes, sometimes seen in stroke survivors.

Hypertension:

High blood pressure, a major stroke risk factor.

Hypertensive Crisis:

A severe spike in blood pressure.

Hypertensive Encephalopathy:

Brain dysfunction due to severely high blood pressure.

Hypertonia:

Increased muscle tone, leading to stiffness or spasticity.

Hyperventilation:

Rapid and shallow breathing, often causing a decrease in carbon dioxide levels.

Hypoglossal Nerve:

The nerve that controls tongue movement and speech.

Hypotension:

Low blood pressure.

Hypothermia:

Abnormally low body temperature, which can be a complication after a stroke.

Hypotonic:

Having decreased muscle tone.

Hypovolemic Shock:

A life-threatening condition due to low blood volume.

Infarct:

Tissue death due to a lack of blood supply.

Interventional Radiologist:

A specialist who performs minimally invasive procedures using imaging guidance.

Intracerebral Haemorrhage:

Bleeding within the brain tissue.

Intracerebral Haematoma:

A collection of blood within the brain tissue.

Intracerebral:

Inside the brain tissue.

Intracranial Aneurysm:

A bulge or weak spot in a blood vessel inside the brain.

Intracranial Atherosclerosis:

Narrowing of blood vessels within the brain.

Intracranial Haemorrhage (ICH):

Bleeding within the skull, often seen in haemorrhagic strokes.

Intracranial Pressure (ICP):

Pressure inside the skull, which can rise after a stroke.

Intracranial Pressure Monitoring:

Measurement of pressure within the skull.

Intracranial Stenosis:

Narrowing of blood vessels within the brain.

Intrathecal:

Within the spinal canal.

Intravenous (IV) Line:

A tube used to deliver fluids or medication directly into a vein.

Intravenous (IV) Push:

Rapid administration of medication directly into a vein.

Intravenous Thrombolysis:

Administering clot-dissolving medication through an IV.

Intubation:

Placement of a tube into the airway to assist with breathing.

Irrigational Therapy:

Cleaning and flushing of wounds or body cavities.

Ischemic Cascade:

A series of events leading to tissue damage during an ischemic stroke.

Ischemic Penumbra:

Brain tissue at risk of damage due to reduced blood flow.

Ischemic Stroke:

A blockage in a blood vessel leading to the brain, often caused by a blood clot.

Laryngectomy:

Surgical removal of the larynx (voice box).

Laryngopharynx:

The part of the throat where the airway and digestive tract meet.

Laryngoscopy:

A procedure to examine the larynx and vocal cords.

Laryngospasm:

A sudden, involuntary closure of the vocal cords, causing difficulty breathing.

Leukoaraiosis:

White matter changes in the brain, often associated with small vessel disease.

Lipid Profile:

Blood test results indicating cholesterol levels.

Motor Cortex:

The part of the brain responsible for controlling movement.

Motor Skills:

Abilities related to movement and coordination.

MRI (Magnetic Resonance Imaging):

A scan that provides detailed images of the brain.

Myelin

The protective covering of nerve fibres.

Myocardial Infarction (Heart Attack):

Damage to the heart muscle due to reduced blood flow.

Myoclonic Seizures:

Sudden, brief muscle jerks.

Myoclonus:

Sudden, involuntary muscle jerks.

Myopathy:

A disorder of the muscles.

Nasal Cannula:

A device used to deliver oxygen through the nostrils.

Nasogastric (NG) Tube Feeding:

Nutritional support is delivered via a tube through the nose and into the stomach.

Nasogastric Tube:

A tube inserted through the nose into the stomach for feeding or medication.

Nebuliser Medication:

Liquid medication converted into a fine mist for inhalation.

Nebuliser:

A device that delivers medication in a fine mist form for inhalation.

Neurogenic Bladder:

A condition where nerve damage affects bladder control.

Neurogenic Bowel:

Bowel dysfunction due to nerve damage.

Neurogenic Shock:

A type of shock resulting from nervous system dysfunction.

Neurogenic Shock:

Shock resulting from nervous system dysfunction.

Neuroimaging:

Techniques to visualise the brain's structure and function.

Neurointerventionalist:

A specialist in minimally invasive treatments for neurological conditions.

Neurological Assessment:

Evaluation of the nervous system's function.

Neurological Deficit:

A problem with the nervous system, often seen after a stroke.

Neurological Rehabilitation:

Therapy to improve brain function and mobility.

Neurologist:

A doctor who specialises in treating disorders of the nervous system, including strokes.

Neuroplasticity:

The brain's ability to adapt and reorganise after injury.

Neuroprotective:

Interventions to protect brain tissue from further damage.

Neuropsychological Assessment:

Evaluation of cognitive function after a stroke.

Neuropsychologist:

A specialist who assesses cognitive functions and behaviour.

Neurotransmitter:

Chemicals in the brain that transmit messages between nerve cells.

Neurotrophic:

Promoting the growth and development of nerve cell

Oral Motor Exercises:

Activities to improve mouth and tongue movement for

speech and swallowing.

Orthopaedic Surgeon:

A doctor specialising in the treatment of bone and joint conditions.

Orthostatic Hypotension:

A sudden drop in blood pressure when changing position.

Oxygen Saturation:

A measure of the oxygen-carrying capacity of the blood.

Oxygen Therapy:

The administration of oxygen to improve oxygen levels in the blood.

Palliative Care:

Supportive care focused on symptom relief and improving quality of life.

Paraesthesia:

Abnormal sensations, such as tingling or numbness.

Paraplegia:

Paralysis affecting the lower half of the body.

Perfusion Deficit:

Inadequate blood flow to tissues, including the brain.

Peripheral Artery Disease (PAD):

Narrowing of blood vessels outside the heart and brain.

Peripheral Neuropathy:

Nerve damage affecting extremities, sometimes linked to stroke.

Peripherally Inserted Central Catheter (PICC):

A long, thin tube inserted into a vein for intravenous therapy.

Pneumonia:

Infection or inflammation of the lungs, a potential complication after a stroke.

Post-Stroke Fatigue:

An overwhelming sense of tiredness or exhaustion that often affects stroke survivors. It can be a persistent and challenging symptom, making daily activities more difficult.

Pulmonary Edema:

Fluid build-up in the lungs.

Pulmonary Embolism:

A blood clot in the lung, a potential complication of stroke.

Pulmonary Function Test:

A lung function test to assess breathing capacity.

Pulmonary Rehabilitation:

A program to improve lung function after a stroke.

Pulmonary Toilet:

Techniques to clear mucus and secretions from the airways.

Pulse Oximetry:

A device to measure oxygen levels in the blood.

Rehabilitation Engineer:

An expert who designs assistive devices for stroke survivors.

Rehabilitation:

Therapy to regain lost skills and functions after a stroke.

Respiratory Therapist:

A healthcare professional who specialises in treating breathing problems.

Risk Factor:

Something that increases the chance of having a stroke.

Saccade:

Rapid eye movement from one point to another.

Sensorimotor:

Involving both sensory and motor functions.

Sialorrhea:

Excessive drooling, sometimes seen in stroke patients.

Spasticity:

Muscle stiffness or tightness, often seen in stroke patients.

Speech Therapist:

A professional who helps with speech and communication difficulties.

Spinal Tap (Lumbar Puncture):

A procedure to collect cerebrospinal fluid for testing.

Statins:

Medications to lower cholesterol levels and reduce stroke risk.

Sternal Precautions:

Restrictions on certain movements after chest surgery.

Stroke Unit:

A specialised hospital unit for stroke patients' care and monitoring.

Stoma:

An opening surgically created in the body, such as a tracheostomy stoma.

Subarachnoid Haemorrhage:

Bleeding in the space surrounding the brain.

Subarachnoid Space:

The space between the brain and the surrounding membrane.

Subdural Haemorrhage:

Bleeding between the brain's surface and its outer covering.

Subdural Haematoma:

Bleeding between the brain and its outer covering.

Sublingual Medication:

Medication placed under the tongue for rapid absorption.

Tachycardia:

Abnormally fast heartbeat.

Tachycardic:

Having a heart rate that is faster than normal.

Tachypnoea:

Rapid breathing.

Thrombectomy:

A procedure to remove a clot from a blood vessel.

Thrombocytopenia:

A condition characterised by low platelet counts, leading to increased bleeding risk.

Thrombocytopenia:

A low platelet count, which can increase bleeding risk.

Thrombocytosis:

Elevated platelet levels, which can increase stroke risk.

Thrombolysis:

Treatment to break down blood clots.

Thrombolytic Agent:

Medication used to dissolve blood clots.

Thrombolytic Therapy:

Treatment to break down blood clots, often using tPA.

Thrombophilia:

A tendency to develop blood clots, which can be a stroke risk factor.

Tinnitus:

Ringing or buzzing in the ears, which can be a symptom of a stroke.

Tissue Plasminogen Activator (tPA):

Medication used to dissolve blood clots.

Tracheostomy Care:

Maintenance and cleaning of the tracheostomy site and tube.

Tracheostomy:

A surgical procedure to create an opening in the windpipe for breathing.

Transient Ischemic Attack (TIA):

Sometimes called a "mini-stroke," it's a temporary blockage of blood flow to the brain with no lasting damage.

Tremor:

Involuntary shaking, which can occur in stroke survivors.

Vascular Bypass Surgery:

A procedure to create a new route for blood flow, often used in stroke prevention.

Vascular Dementia:

Cognitive decline due to impaired blood flow in the brain.

Vascular Graft:

A surgically implanted tube used to replace or repair a blood vessel.

Vascular Risk Factors:

Factors related to the health of blood vessels, affecting stroke risk.

Vasodilator Medications:

Drugs that widen blood vessels, increasing blood flow.

Vasospasm:

Narrowing of blood vessels, potentially causing reduced blood flow.

Vaso spasticity:

Abnormal narrowing of blood vessels.

Venous Access Device:

A catheter placed into a vein for medical treatments, such as IV medications.

Venous Duplex Ultrasound:

A test to evaluate blood flow in veins.

Venous Sinus Thrombosis:

Blood clot in the brain's venous sinuses, a rare cause of stroke.

Venous Thromboembolism (VTE):

Blood clots in the veins, which can be a complication of stroke.

Ventilator:

A machine that assists with breathing when the lungs are compromised.

Ventricular Drain:

A tube inserted into the brain to relieve pressure or drain excess fluid.

Ventriculostomy:

Surgical creation of an opening in a brain ventricle.

Vertigo:

A sensation of spinning or dizziness.

Vocal Cord Paralysis:

Loss of movement in one or both vocal cords.

About the Author

The author's life took an unexpected turn at 46 when a devastating stroke in 2011 reshaped his world.

Navigating the physical and emotional aftermath of stroke, largely on his own, the author intimately understood the daily unspoken struggles that both survivors and caregivers face. He experienced firsthand the immense burden placed on unprepared family members, many of whom navigate the demanding 24/7 caregiving role without any guidance.

The complexities only deepened when narcissism entered the mix, turning an already challenging situation into an emotional battleground.

With little support and an uncertain future, he found healing through journaling.

Determined to share his hard-earned wisdom, the authors debut book—The Stroke Survivor HandBook—was first published in 2016. A simple act that blossomed into a new passion as an author, and he now dedicates his writing to offering practical advice, emotional support, and hope to stroke survivors, caregivers, and those dealing with narcissism.

His books are a lifeline for anyone facing these trials, providing readers with the tools to navigate their toughest moments and find strength in the face of adversity.

Share Your Experience

Dear Esteemed Reader,

Thank you sincerely for choosing my book during this challenging time. I'm truly honoured that you've decided to embark on this journey with me. Your trust fills me with deep gratitude and a renewed sense of purpose as I share these insights and support with you.

As you explore this handbook, I hope you find insights that resonate, guidance that supports you, and stories that inspire strength and resilience. Your experience as a reader is invaluable, and I would be honoured if you could spare a moment to share your thoughts.

Reviews are the lifeblood of any writer's career. They provide invaluable feedback and help guide other readers in discovering this book. Whether you choose to share a brief sentiment or a detailed analysis, your honest opinion holds great significance.

If you found this book helpful, please consider leaving a review on the platform where you obtained it. Your support in spreading the word would be immensely appreciated.

Conversely, if the book did not meet your expectations, I welcome your constructive criticism. Please feel free to reach out using the contact details provided at the beginning of the book. Such feedback allows me to grow as a writer and create future works that better align with readers' needs.

Once again, I extend my sincerest gratitude for your support. Thank you for allowing me to be part of your journey. Your encouragement means the world to me, and I am deeply grateful to each person who picks up this handbook.

Together, we can build a community of resilience and hope for stroke survivors and their caregivers all over the world.

Warm regards,

Brian Maram

The Stroke Survivor HandBook 2nd ed.

Other Books by Author

Through the Eyes of a Survivor - Stroke

Through the Eyes of a Survivor-Traumatic Brain Injury

Narcissism - The Face in the Mirror

Starter Book: Stroke Activity Puzzles (Menda Brain)

Intermediate Book: Stroke Activity Puzzles (Menda Brain)

Advanced Book: Stroke Activity Puzzles (Menda Brain)

www.neuvare.com

www.ingramcontent.com/pod-product-compliance
Lightning Source LLC
Chambersburg PA
CBHW071348150726
47997CB00002B/900